Simple Wellness

By Samantha Durland, M.D.

As told to Barbara Warner, Ph.D.

Simple Wellness by Samantha Durland, M.D.

As told to Barbara Warner, Ph.D.

Cover design by Barbara Burket
Printed by CreateSpace, an Amazon.com company

First soft cover edition 2018

1. Durland, Samantha, M.D. 2. Physicians – United States Self-Help (Health and Fitness) I. Simple Wellness

Dedication

I dedicate this book to Brandon, my husband and sweetheart, for loving me for who I am, for allowing me to take this path and for teaching me to stand up for myself. To my boys, know that every day I am thankful to be your mom. To my grandfather, Gaylord Neighbor, thank you for teaching me love of the human body and the value of hard work. And for everyone else along the way, thank you for … well … everything. This book would not have existed without your help.

"Success is no accident. It is hard work, perseverance, learning, studying, sacrifice and, most of all, love of what you are doing or learning to do."

- Edson Arantes do Nascimento, also known as Pelé, retired Brazilian professional footballer

"In times of stress, the best thing we can do for each other is to listen with our ears and our hearts and to be assured that our questions are just as important as our answers."

- Fred Rogers, "The World According to Mister Rogers: Important Things to Remember"

Table of Contents

It's Okay

It's okay to believe
It's okay to cry
It's okay to laugh
It's okay to feel sorrow
It's okay to feel joy
It's okay to not be sure
It's okay to be yourself
It's okay to just be

We are all here for a reason
We all have a story

If we spend our whole life wanting to be someone else, we miss who we are
If we spend our whole life thinking about tomorrow, we forget to see everything about today
If we think we have to figure it all out, we are thinking from our head and not our hearts ... we miss the point and all the messages on the way

Open your eyes and you will see
Open your heart, and you will feel
Listen and you will hear
Take a deep breath
You will see ... it has never left you
It has always been there
It already is
You already are
It is all around you, and it always has been

You have nothing to prove
It has already been proven

Listen…See…Feel…
It's okay

Chapter 1

Introduction

My patients call me Sam. That's because I don't just think of myself as their medical doctor. I am at my core a human being like them, as well as a wife, a mother and a doctor.

My wellness journey has led me to a combination of holistic and classic medicine in a practice that is growing today. I want to share that journey with you because it helps explain my approach to my patients and to others who I see as fellow travelers on this wonderful journey we call life. I believe that together, as we learn from each other, we can be empowered to make our lives better. Together we can overcome our fear of our bodies and partner with them, thinking of them as our dear friends that love us and want only what is best for us.

So really, this book is about you.

Our aging bodies are the carriers of our maturing eternal spirit, the part of us that makes us who we are, the part of us that is wired seamlessly into our being. Our bodies are the product of thousands of years of genetic adaptation, which I call our basic genetic rule book, also known as our DNA. They are always working to help us, not go against us, because they are the embodiment of nature. And nature wants what is best for us. In fact, nature wants us to be well our whole life.

However, we have put our bodies under tremendous stress in our society, chronically elevating our stress hormones so that we are more subject to illness and to the production of unhealthy fat. As a result, our body's natural ability to regenerate itself, no matter what our age, has been stressed. And our regenerative system has become confused. We have forgotten the simple precepts that govern wellness. And classic, or conventional, medicine has not always helped us.

But my belief, borne out of years of experience, is that if we give our systems energy, we can regain that regenerative capacity that has served us so well and that is built into our genetic rule book.

When we focus on giving the body energy, we allow it to do whatever it wants to do, and that is to correct itself. We get to the heart of the problem. We don't just focus on lowering the cholesterol – we focus on finding out why it's elevated and try to correct the problem. Only then can true healing occur.

My belief in the perfecting nature of our bodies has proven itself over and over again in my years in practice and in my own personal life. I like to get to the "why" of things, rather than just try to manage symptoms primarily through medications. But that doesn't mean there isn't a time for classic medicine. We just have to know when we need to turn to it as part of a larger holistic model.

So, my main goal is to tune in to that primal energy in the body. And it is this desire that now distinguishes my practice. I am taking my classic training and moving beyond it to embody all that I know to be true about wellness. And I am applying it to all ages and genders.

For the first 25 or so years of our life, we are "hardwiring" our bodies around our spirit, much as one might program a computer. The input is our experiences, our perceptions, our understanding, our emotions, our value systems, our treatment of ourselves, our identities, our aspirations, our framework for decision-making, our community, our role models, our genetic makeup, how we play, what we eat, and so much more. We learn what it feels like to be in balance and what it feels like to be out of balance. Hopefully during this time we get our first life lessons in being intentional about our body's environment. And during this time we usually have plenty of natural bodily energy to expend.

During these crucial years of psyche formation we learn stress responses (around age 5). Stress responses are keyed to the release of the hormone cortisol, which is uncomfortable to experience. We learn to either hold on to the stress (internalize it) or give it away (externalize it), or a combination of both.

By age 25 or so, the frontal lobe of our brain is mature, or at least less "ignorant." And around ages 35 to 40, the body starts the aging process. The impact of life has more effect at that point because there is less natural energy. This can be a confusing time because we may still want to try to expend the same amount of energy as we did when we were young, expecting the same level of recovery. But if you do tip the balance and push against your genetic rule book, you can get sick – because it takes energy you no longer have.

But all is not lost beyond those first 25 years. Your body forgives you for the mistakes you have made, including subjecting it to too much stress. Your brain cannot change your genes, but it can work with them. There is always a workaround if you play by the basic rules of wellness.

You can still rewire/reprogram your brain to a large extent as it relates to disease and injury because the brain has what we call positive neuroplasticity, meaning that it can make new connections. It just takes the desire (how you think) and the energy (in the body) to do so. It needs the energy to pull out the old connection and the intent to plug in the new one.

I love helping people change how they think and find the energy to put that new thinking into action. In fact, I don't believe in the adage that you can't teach an old dog new tricks. Give that dog a little energy, and it can do anything.

Our system does have a breaking point, however. It will sacrifice a lot of other functions to keep the brain and the heart working. It can get confused and turn against itself unintentionally, sometimes resulting in an autoimmune disease, where the body turns against itself. While classic medicine can play a role in helping the body deal with such disease states, it does not have all the answers. That's why we need to better connect with our body's needs and reenergize it. We need to unlearn the fear and chronic stress that has hurt our bodies.

With that in mind, I strive to help people listen to their bodies, to think of their lives differently and to realize that they are healthier than they think – and can be healthier than they fear. I believe we all have this ability within us, and when we tap into it amazing things will happen in our bodies and in our lives.

In essence, I help people understand their body's response to stress and how to energize themselves to better deal with stress. This adjustment helps them stay healthier and gives their lives more meaning. It helps them live in the present. It helps them sit in the driver's seat of their bodies and their life, rather than feel like they are simply on a survival treadmill.

I help people listen to their body and make better decisions that reflect its wishes. I help them get more in touch with themselves and in essence become their own healers.

In short, I help them actually enjoy the journey of life.

While we all share a human makeup, we are all unique. I am a guide, a voice for the story that your body is telling you, in the context of the human rule book by which we all operate.

I hope this book will help you better translate your body's messages so that you can be more mindful, see more meaning and acquire a brighter perspective about your journey. I hope you learn to love the miracle that is your body and to establish, or reestablish, a more robust stress response that does not control you – instead you control and respect it.

As part of this process, I've developed a Simple 7 framework of reference for how to treat your body so that you can do this. I unify biology and psychology, considering them equally important and wholly intertwined. And I do this with a team of people who help support this process.

Why do I do this? I am drawn to helping people finding peace within themselves. It lifts me up and rejuvenates me. For me, helping people is vital to my wellbeing. And when people find peace, they find the energy to live their lives more fully and to help others do the same.

My goal is to help you address elevated stress hormones that can cause the mind to lower its defenses, become much more aware of pain and become more fearful. The mind wants to avoid pain at all costs, especially chronic pain, which fatigues both the body and the mind. We need to energize our brain, our control center, and relieve the stress by going back to the simple things that empower us: reenergizing ourselves, taking in the right elements, finding self-esteem, eating properly, achieving a sense of equilibrium, eliminating toxins and engaging in community. These are my Simple 7 ways to thrive in a strong, healthy, peaceful body.

When we return to the basic rule book (our primal nature), we learn to self-correct what is self-induced, to put a stop to the cycle of sickness, to re-teach our bodies to undo the damage, to better control the way we think about wellness and to reduce stress. The brain can then relax, help us reconnect with wellness and figure out what we are meant to do in this world. We help the body find energy to heal itself.

And so, this is primarily a book about loving ourselves, following our genetic rule book, allowing our bodies to release stress and find energy, and rebooting our natural regenerative capacity, no matter what our age, no matter what our gender.

I will share with you my background and my personal evolution toward this wellness model. I will outline for you my philosophy of wellness. I will discuss the premises of wellness by which I operate and give tips on how to reduce stress and find energy. And I will outline my Simple 7 solution to wellness.

Let me start by sharing a bit of my background so that you understand what brought me to the beliefs that empower my evolving wellness practice.

Chapter 2

My Personal Wellness Evolution

I want to tell you how I arrived at my philosophy of wellness that I practice today. And the more I think about it, it all began in my childhood, when I decided I wanted to be the best I could be.

It was in the first grade that I realized I could match the intellectual abilities of the "gifted" students simply by studying harder. In fact, I am only now learning that spending four hours a day on homework in the seventh grade is not normal – but I did it over and over again, with the goal of being the best.

During my elementary- and middle-school years, I learned to appreciate movement and nature, as each summer I rode horses, hiked and backpacked at a camp in Colorado. I began to love activity. I learned to appreciate the awe-inspiring beauty of nature. And I began to get a larger picture of what I would become in the midst of all this greatness and beauty.

I was lucky. I had a good family and home life. I came to believe that life was wonderful and that I should be thankful every day. Still, life wasn't one long, positive trajectory upward. But here's the key: Instead of thinking the cup was half empty, I intentionally determined that it was half full. And over time, my mind believed this. That positive outlook would come to influence the evolution of my medical practice to be what it is today.

In high school, I graduated first in my class. And I graduated from college in three years. I began to believe that if there is something you want to do, you can do it. And I began to see how I could support others in their goals. I realized that if I could do it, anyone could.

My grandfather had been a doctor, and I decided I wanted to go to medical school too, so I could take care of people. And there I adopted the same mindset I did in first grade when I realized I could be a "gifted" student. The first year of medical school was fast-paced, condensed and jam-packed with information. I started wondering if it was doable. Then one day I saw more than 130 second-year medical students leave an auditorium and realized that if they could make it through their first year, I could also. It was a matter of working hard and believing in myself.

As the retired Brazilian professional footballer, Pelé, once said, "Success is no accident. It is hard work, perseverance, learning, studying, sacrifice and most of all love of what you are doing or learning to do." And I began to live that more fully.

I attended medical school at the University of Kansas Medical Center, graduating in 1999. I then chose an obstetrics and gynecology residency at the University of Iowa and at the KU Medical Center, graduating from my residency in 2003. I chose obstetrics and gynecology (OB-GYN) as my specialty because I loved talking with people and figuring things out. It was a mix of everything, including learning how the body worked.

I was in group private practice with OB-GYN specialists at a local hospital for just over 12 years before moving to a private practice in 2015 as a general practitioner/OB-GYN specialist. During the last years of group practice, I became board certified in anti-aging and regenerative medicine through the American Academy of Anti-Aging Medicine. I also did a fellowship in metabolic and nutritional medicine through the Metabolic Medical Institute.

I became confident in my practice of medicine. I understood the system and the importance of working as a team. I was employed and financially okay. I was "successful" in my group practice. But I felt a higher calling to a better way. So, I quit and followed my heart. And that's brought me to where I am today.

In classic practice, I realized there was much I did not have control over, including the stunning uniqueness of our individual nature. And I realized that the classic practice of medicine could not conquer all ills. I did, however, have the ability to help patients through difficult experiences. And I found that when I started sharing my humanity with them – crying with them, hugging them and emphasizing to them they were not alone – that I was being who I was supposed to be – a person with a sense of humanity and a faith in the power of nature to make things right. I would give them permission that was not necessarily mine to give (but which made them feel less alone) to do what they had to do, to find peace, to believe in themselves and to keep going.

But that's not what I was taught.

I had taken vows in medical school to do no harm. But I wasn't sure classic medicine was enabling me to help them. The patients I was seeing looked sad. The system did not allow time to deal with the real issues. I could not see all my patients and get all the work done within that system. There was no time to properly educate my patients and be part of their lives. There was no balance.

I noticed that as doctors we were talking a lot about prevention. Yet we were focused on disease, as if the body was a vortex of illness that we could not help make well. We were blind as to why people were becoming sicker. At the same time, I had a growing knowledge that the body does not want to be sick. Its job is to protect us, as it does when it fends off viruses to which it has built up immunity.

It began to settle in me that one of the main problems people were facing was chronic stress, which was not only injuring the body but also the mind. The body cannot heal in this state. It is depleted. Over time, as we over-tax our energy reserves, we start to feel more pain, find it hard to think or sleep, feel slower, seek out the quick fix of sugar, or try to dissociate ourselves from our mind and body by drinking, smoking or other means. And when we don't feel well for a long time and cannot understand why, the brain stops trying. Pretty soon we are on the couch all the time eating potato chips and don't know how we got there. But what we don't always understand is that if we just replenish our body's energy, it can recover its never-ending regenerative ability. Just because we let our reserve tanks get low doesn't mean the body can't fix itself – if it has the energy to do so.

The chronically stressful industrialized world we have created is not what our body understands. Our body is primal. It just wants us to eat whole foods, drink water, sleep, feel a sense of value, connect with community, take care of its digestive system and move. It could care less about the size of the home that we live in or the car we drive. It just wants the consistency of a good day.

We cannot overcome these basic needs no matter what we think. Our primal nature is encrypted in our genetic rule book, our DNA. And once we accept this and return to that basic path, we become healthier.

In my classic practice, I had been doing the opposite. I was spending hours each day seeing patients, only to go home to put my children to bed and then go back to the hospital for evening baby deliveries. I experienced many life and death situations. In between, I got whatever sleep I could get. I would return home in the morning to start all over again. I was on a never-ending hamster wheel – I was giving to everyone, but at the expense of my body. And as I aged my body couldn't tolerate that level of output. I felt like I was drowning every day.

I started having anxiety issues and found myself crying on the way to work one day. I was not delivering the level of care that I wanted. A part of me was dying, and it was the important part, the part that had set me apart. The life I was living was not healthy or sustainable. I remember that this revelation hit me at 4:30 p.m. on a Friday afternoon. I thought to myself that I could go broke if I left what I was doing. But the alternative was to feel dead inside. And so, I made the decision that I would not die, that my ultimate sadness and despair meant I was not being true to myself. And I decided to transition to a different way of practicing medicine.

My break from my old group partners was not a happy one. Our relationship had always seemed sound. But apparently, I had become their competition. While I continued to live in the same community, the day I left they said they would not back me up on surgical privileges. That meant that I could have lost my ability to perform operations simply because I was no longer their partner, not because of any lack of skills or bad outcomes. This was very hurtful to me. But with time I decided that being irritated with the situation gave energy to something I could not change. If I believed energy was precious (and I did), then giving energy to this irritation was only weakening me. And I had a long journey ahead for which I needed that energy. So, I let go of my irritation. And thanks to the confidence my other colleagues in the medical community had in me, my privileges were restored.

I had thought the transition to my own private classic practice would make things better. But I found that private practice did not solve the problem because of the expense of insurance billing practices. I still couldn't deliver the standard of care I wanted. I was still constrained by a system governed by rules that were not focused on wellness. And I realized that people were not being properly taught or rewarded for taking care of their bodies.

It's important to realize that the health insurance industry is just a third-party vendor that is in the business of dispersing payments for services provided. It's not your doctor. Its job is not wellness. True wellness is an individual choice. But there is so much more to wellness than any one organ system, or all these systems put together – or just treating symptoms without getting to the cause.

Private practice in a classic system was not the answer. When I would see women for a well-woman exam, as permitted by insurance systems, I was limited to a pap test and a pelvic exam. These tests were what were supposed to define wellness. But when I looked into women's eyes as they left my office, they still looked sad. And I didn't feel like I was doing all I could. Under the rules of insurance, I still had to treat patients as if they were all the same. And sometimes my decisions were overruled by insurance managers. I realized once again that what I was doing in the practice of medicine was not working. And I was again breaking right along with it.

I was drawn to provide more solutions to the practice of medicine and patient care. And ultimately that resulted in my break from classic medicine in the confines of a defined medical system, a system that is doing some things right, but doing so many things wrong. And this led to my break from the health insurance system.

I knew this would invite scrutiny. But I also knew I had to do it because I believe that medicine requires not only doing no harm, but also making a meaningful connection with patients. I had to start from the ground level and really get what wellness was all about. I had to find a way to give patients energy and help them reduce their stress.

And despite my tendency to overthink things, I never looked back. I learned to trust that whatever was happening was the way that it is supposed to be. And the more I let it be, the better it got.

It may surprise you to learn that doctors can get scared about what they are asked to do on a daily basis. They don't have all the answers. No one does. But I realized that I could no longer practice from fear. Nor could I treat everyone as if they were the same and focus on symptoms. There I would see only limited healing. While I saw my classic training as valuable, I embraced a lot more. And so I ended up somewhere in the middle between classic and holistic medicine, just a fellow human being who loves to help people get better, who teaches people how to be their best selves. It's that simple.

I quit my private obstetrical practice in 2015 to open my current practice that combines holistic and classic medicine in a way that is free of the complicated and frustrating insurance system. In 2018, I stopped accepting health insurance altogether and went to a pay as you go model. I stopped being governed by the business of insurance and became guided by my own values and principles of wellness. I developed a set price list for my services, striving for transparency. After all, it had always seemed odd to me to think that patients, as consumers, were basically uninformed about how the system works or its pricing mechanism. Insurance companies have cost markups in so many places. And the lack of transparency in the classic medical system is overwhelming. As a result, patients/consumers have difficulty properly evaluating what they are getting for their money. What other type of business operates that way outside of medicine?

Nevertheless, people in the medical system thought I was crazy for choosing this model. Why would someone who was financially secure quit a successful practice? But in my eyes, I was not successful any more. And certainly, being between holistic and classic medicine can be isolating because the two are unfortunately so often at odds. But I know both have value, and I have come to a place of peace on this.

During this whole professional transformation, I was also undergoing a personal one. It took me several years to mentally and physically get where I am, to feel like my body was in balance. And now I realize that there is no static balance. Instead we need to constantly listen to our body and adjust our lives as needed. It is the willingness to do so that sets us apart.

In those years of learning to listen to my body I started eating whole foods in frequent, small meals. I ate items lower on the glycemic scale, which meant eating fewer carbohydrates and other foods that process quickly in the body and can lead to spikes in blood glucose levels that affect insulin levels. I moderated my exercise. Too little exercise and things don't work well – and we are more tired. But too much exercise is stressful to the body and can break it down.

I also learned to overcome fear of my physical body. And here competitive amateur boxing was helpful. I found boxing was not only a great stress reliever but also a game of chess and opposing wills. It was an opportunity to look fear in the face and fight back. Fear gives too much energy away and weakens us. In boxing, I learned to pace myself, letting go in bursts and allowing for recovery.

I ended up with my own exercise model that includes weightlifting, amateur boxing, cardiovascular work and simply moving, knowing that muscles tighten with age. That's not to say I did it all perfectly. But I developed a sustainable, consistent journey. When I fell off the wagon, I started again the next day – no guilt.

All this and more I have applied to my newly evolving practice, which incorporates the best tools of classic and holistic medicine, that treats both men and women of all ages and has a special focus on aging. It is by living this journey myself that I came to understand it.

I now apply my medical school, personal and holistic training to what I know about wellness so that patients can maximize their healing potential and actually start to feel well. It is so rewarding to see a return of that spark in their eyes.

I have come to realize that if you build a practice based upon the principles of the mind, body and spirit, people will come. They are hungry for this in these days of dehumanization. They want to be well. And they want it to be simple.

Chapter 3
My Philosophy of Wellness

My journey toward wellness for myself and my patients has been built upon core beliefs that grew out of my personal experience and objective data from my years of practice, patient feedback and the results I have repeatedly seen.

In the process, I have compiled a database containing laboratory results and measurements of body composition and other factors, to which I frequently refer and update.

My approach to wellness is to first practice from the standpoint of love because I believe that love is the strongest and most healing energy of all. It is pure. It fills the body with amazing power. It conquers fear. It is the best medicine. And by looking through the eyes of love at a patient I can see so much more.

When I look at patients with love, it becomes apparent to me the reasons they do not feel well. I sit and listen to their stories and their experiences. I learn their belief system. I let them know I am there for them and will never judge them. I look into their eyes and realize how awesome they are. I help them overcome their fear and become empowered.

By combining my training, my accumulated data, my listening and my simple caring, I am able to see more clearly the answers to people's wellness problems. I am better able to help people rewire their bodies to be who they truly were meant to be. And in the process, I become who I truly was meant to be. I can more clearly see now what it is that I do best. And I can teach and empower others.

I have listened to hundreds of people tell me about their lives. I love taking the time to do this because it enables me to take better care of them. As I come to understand the source of their stress, I can start to untangle their wellness problems with a combination of herbal, mindful and physical prescriptions. I help them reconnect with the best parts of themselves so they can increase the quality of their lives.

I make my decisions for myself and others without ruminating, which just adds doubt and saps energy. I think for a couple of days about an issue, then choose the peaceful path that feels right. I find that my competitive nature is an advantage, just as it was in my youth and during medical school. I am always studying others because I like to win – for myself and for my patients. I can be relentless and driven in the cause of greater wellness. And I am determined to remain intense and genuine.

I want people to get better, but I have to know they are willing to fight for that, that they are willing to try to achieve wellness. I won't sink with them (lest we sink together), but I will float with them until they signal they want help and I can pull them up on the raft along with me. As long as they keep trying, I will stay with them until they develop their own sense of self.

I would say that my philosophy of simple wellness boils down to this: Our body houses our eternal spirit. It is built to protect that spirit from the day we were created until the day it dies. It is one with us. It will sacrifice itself for the sake of the spirit's journey. But it has a set amount of physical energy for us to use as we like. So the energy balance between us and the world around us is crucial to our health. Our wellness is never nature versus nurture or just a bunch of laboratory results; it is more than that, including our genetics, how we grew up, our life events, the way we deal with stress, how we process emotions and so much more. Wellness has to be seen through the eyes of the body, the protector of the spiritual self. The body is our warrior and our best friend, not our enemy. If we listen, the body talks. It tells us what to do to get back to wellness.

Before our body focuses on our well-being, however, its first concern is survival. And the rule book it uses for this is more than 100,000 years of genetic adaption, our genetic code or DNA. It is the primal core of us. It is the way our body has evolved to survive biological stressors.

As a result, our body makes decisions from an energy perspective. It asks, What is the most efficient way to keep us alive, to give us a survival benefit? How can it help us navigate this world safely? How does it get the most return for the least expenditure of energy? How can we regenerate ourselves? Our body will even hide things that are wrong from us before we know anything has happened, as it tries to heal itself. And if it perceives danger, it will run. Or in the case of chronic stress, it will lie down and stop moving to conserve energy.

Although we are highly evolved, we have not evolved beyond our body's basic rule book. Yet society has changed so much that it is constantly over-stressing that rule book, oftentimes beyond our body's capacity to maintain wellness. We live in a world of too many situational stressors and an abundance of electronics that separate us and cause us to stop moving. As we try to modernize our world, we are mentally trying to evolve faster than our body and nature allow. This does damage to the spirit. We must, therefore, work within our genetic rule book. We must embrace our primal code and work with it rather than against it.

Diseases such as diabetes, high cholesterol, thyroid problems, gastrointestinal (GI) issues, obesity and a host of others, are on the rise. But I think we are just messing up our body's compensatory mechanisms through the stresses of the society we have created. And if we only address these specific diseases, we are missing something. Everything is related. If we give the body back its ability to fix things, it can do an amazing job. Then, if there is still some pathology left behind, we can address that both holistically and through classic medicine.

I always start the wellness journey with a patient's belief system, whether that be holistic or classic, or a combination of both. Then we look at what's causing the stress. I find that if we can fix people's stressors, their bodies can heal themselves. I learn what's going on in people's lives and what they hope to achieve. I then obtain any objective data I need through tests. I ask the body where it is "off."

In follow-up appointments, we examine the objective data and discuss the physical and emotional stresses. Together we come up with a long-term plan for achieving balance. We work on alleviating the stressors to help people's bodies correct metabolic inefficiencies (hormonal, thyroid and insulin imbalances, all of which can affect body composition). And if we do as much as we can and the problems remain, we turn to more classic approaches.

This brings us to a discussion of the importance of energy in the regeneration process. It is important to believe that our body never loses its regenerative capacity. But we must abide by the language of its rule book – what it can and cannot take, what it does and does not want – in order to help it heal itself. To regenerate, to change our hardwired connections, we need energy. And I'm not just talking food here, although that is part of it. We need a connection with the life force both within and without. We have to intentionally build a healthier stress response to break the cycle and find energy. We have to understand and connect with one another – learn to see things through each other's eyes – if we want this to work best. Our interconnectedness is crucial to our energy because we share the common bond of our human nature, while also remaining unique individuals.

I find that most patients dealing with problems are highly stressed, often situationally or emotionally. Bottled-up stress can become a toxic energy that causes the body to become inflamed and break down, even if that stress is simply the processing of thoughts.

I like to think of the stress response as either rhino or bear in nature. The "rhino" response is often easier to address because it is acute or short-term. I equate it to patients feeling like they're running from a rhinoceros. They are anxious and jittery, feeling like they have to move all the time. They have trouble sleeping and concentrating. They have a lowered libido. Their acute stress response tells them to run away from something. I help them identify that something and change it so they don't move into what I call a chronic "bear" state.

Those patients in the chronic stress state, and there are far too many of them, usually come to me with their energy depleted. They are like a bear in hibernation. They often have been in this response for some time, and it has taken a toll on their minds, bodies and spirits. They are usually depressed. They may come to me saying they can't lose weight, no matter what they do. They may have low self-esteem. We figure out what gives them energy, so they can get out of this state. But they have to be intentional and consistent in their efforts. Recovery takes time, so they need to be patient, listening to their body as to how fast it can recover. They must pay attention to the need for rest and relaxation, while at the same time making sure they keep physically moving, even in small ways, because the body craves motion.

My job is to help people identify why their bodies are perceiving such ongoing stress and try to correct that imbalance. Once we do this, the body often can shed fat by the simple formula of calories in-calories out, diet and exercise – nature's basic formula that so eluded them before. People learn to feed themselves better. They are no longer at war with their bodies. They've broken an unhealthy stress cycle. Their mind, body and spirit are unified, and they are able to listen to their body's language better.

In essence, I help people understand the rules their body wants to live by, according to its genetic predispositions, and coach them on how to follow that rule book. I teach them how to release themselves from chronic stress so they can again find their energy to live life. I help them shore up their weakened defenses, optimizing their body's regenerative capacity. I help them modify their lifestyles. I operate from the principle that the body is built to heal, is resilient and is powerful.

My goal is to do this simply, with as few tools as possible. I've found a regime of multiple supplements is not sustainable. We are more primal than this. The body doesn't recognize complexity as true wellness. If it did, we would not have evolved from caves and outlived the dinosaurs, developing our adaptive genetic rule book.

The work I do is about simple processes, simple pricing, simple laboratory tests, personalized service, quick attention, easy explanations, treating people well and modernizing medicine to help people de-stress. In doing this, I help set people on the road to positive outcomes and wellness.

Aging and Wellness

I see many people when they are aging, a time that provides a wonderful opportunity to grow, mature and experience life.

However, although we are born to have a buffer against all the stress and toxin buildup, that buffer is finite. As the body ages, we can use up that buffer.

Our eternal spirit matures, but our body ages. This is hard to reconcile. But aging provides an opportunity to restore our body's regenerative capacity, to restore balance, to give back to the body that has carried us for so long.

As we age, we experience oxidative stress. Just like a car rusts over time from exposure to the elements, so does our body produce free radicals as it processes the oxygen we breathe, which allows our cells to produce energy. These free radicals can stress the components of other cells and our genetic structure. The damage can especially affect organs that are the heaviest users of oxygen – the heart, the lungs and the brain. In fact, oxidative stress is suspected as a key component of aging itself.

Our spirits, being timeless, have a hard time recognizing this oxidative process. We may experience sexual dysfunction, wrinkles, fat accumulation and fatigue. And so we may resist aging. But it's important not to dissociate from our body at this time. We should not fear aging or feel alone. Aging is happening to all of us. Now is the time to be innovative and to hold tight to the belief that the body never loses its regenerative capacity. We just need to better speak its language. We need to tap into our body's ability to heal. It is amazing.

Aging is also a time to deal with the painful thoughts and feelings that we may have been able to ignore, but which may begin to weigh us down, sap our energy and make us sick. It is a time to face these issues, deal with them and let them go. We must process our emotions and the way our brain responds to stress. We must learn to stop ruminating, which steals energy. In sum, learning to deal with our past in a healthy way becomes a matter of wellness and survival.

I find many of my aging patients are tired and finding it painful to look back on their lives. I sit with them, hold their hand at times, or simply just look them in the eye and tell them that they are not alone, that they are here for a reason and that everything is going to be okay. We find some energy to give, and then we face whatever it is – all with the intention of letting go. Sharing this energy and processing it gives them rest.

Letting go does not mean that we have to accept what has happened as right or wrong. Letting go just means that we value ourselves enough to open our eyes to what is in front of us, that we don't have to run from our past and that we want to redirect the energy toward living. It is amazing how much we can change our mental processing if we have the energy and intent to do so. And as our understanding of our body increases, we lose our fear of it.

Body Composition and Wellness

I want my patients to be the strongest, leanest version of themselves they can be. This may involve fat loss, a term I prefer to weight loss. Fat loss must be intentional because leanness and muscle are perceived as vulnerable states by our genetic rule book, whereas fat accumulation is seen by nature as protective. And yet so many people are simply focused on losing weight. But while the management of weight is important, wellness is more than that. If you are not well in your mind, your body will continually be in protection mode.

While fat can store energy, it does not burn energy. It is just a bank. Meanwhile, nature sees muscle mass as a vulnerability because it burns calories that we might need in times of privation. Body fat is light. It does not burn calories. Muscle is heavy and burns calories. Nature's laws are governed by energy. If your body perceives its balance of energy is off, you likely will see an increase in fat. If you restore the balance of energy, you can see the muscle component increase and the fat component decrease.

If you are accumulating fat, your body is often responding to chronic stress. We need to figure out why and fix it so the yo-yo effect stops. The answer is not starving yourself. That only causes more stress. Your life has to be in balance for your body to allow you to increase muscle and lose fat. Indeed, the body won't even allow you to put on muscle mass unless your life is in balance.

We accumulate subcutaneous fat cells (the squeezable fat just under the skin) in our first 20 years. And at about age 20 the number of those fat cells is set. Women tend to have more of these cells than men because of their hormonal system. These cells can deflate (much like balloons) or vary in size, but their number remains constant.

We can get rid of subcutaneous fat through simple cosmetic processes that actually remove the balloons, if you will, so that they cannot return. This simple body sculpting process in essence pops the fat balloons.

I pay attention to the issue of fat not just for cosmetic sake or because of societal pressures, but because it can indicate an energy imbalance. People are energized as they watch their bodies change. I tell patients all the time that body sculpting is easy – wellness of the mind is the hard part.

The challenge of muscle versus fat is more acute with age because aging further exposes the need for balance (prior to aging we can kind of cheat on the process, to an extent). The older we get, the more important is the balance in mind, body and spirit. Otherwise our body tends to keep increasing fat and reducing muscle mass, no matter how much less we eat and how much more we move. If there is a serious imbalance, our body just eats up more muscle and puts on more layers of fat to protect us. Then we get discouraged about eating less and moving more, and the problem just gets worse.

While I can help remove the fat cells to quicken the process, I know that just changing the outer body does not correct all things because the mind and body are connected. We can change our body and still feel unrest in our mind. We must correct the imbalance.

With all this in mind, let me offer you some pearls of wisdom that summarize my philosophy:

Pearls of Wisdom

1. **Our bodies are the embodiment of nature.** There are human genetic codes, or rules, of nature that we must all respect in order to thrive. When we work within these rules we become more powerful. When we work against them, or try to override them, we push against the power of nature. In my experience, pushing against our genetic code does not work very well (e.g., consistently overworking to exhaustion or eating mostly processed foods). Ultimately, nature seems to win out. But working within the rules of nature can give us amazing power.
2. **Virtually every decision in nature is based upon the principles of energy.** Nature operates mathematically, with no emotion involved. Just as water and electricity flow to where there is least resistance, so the human body functions best when the energy is allowed to flow with the least pushback, including the least expenditure of energy. Processes that are too complex are too hard to sustain because they go against the rules of nature (e.g., fad diets, using more supplements than the body needs). The goal

should be using and giving away less energy than we need in order to allow the body to heal, thrive and ultimately stay alive.

3. **We must adjust our stress responses to live a more healthy life**. When we are in extreme chronic stress, our body tends to override us in order to keep us alive. Out of basic survival, it may stop us in our tracks rather than allowing us to continue living in an unsustainable way. The body's prime directive is to keep us alive. After that it just wants us to have a good day. Once we learn our body's stress response, its capabilities and how we can keep it centered, we can pretty much do what we want (be in the driver's seat). We can harness the energy of nature to lift us up. We just need to adjust our framework of reference to life's challenges.
4. **We are all human, but we are also individual.** We all share the same basic human rule book, but we also are individual in our value systems. We cannot expect others to share our value system. Instead we must realize others' value systems and empathize with them. For instance, if someone solely believes in classic medicine, I don't expect them to wholly jump on board a holistic approach to wellness.
5. **Love gives energy.** Love is powerfully regenerative, second to no other power. We must consciously employ more of it in our personal lives, in our professions and in the way we shape our world.
6. **All things in nature are connected.** Humans, animals, trees, grass, water – we are all linked and intricately connected. We are not islands. What happens to one can have profound impact on others. When we stand with nature, we are energized. When we sit in a room with a computer, there is minimal connection and no rejuvenation of energy. Without connection life does not thrive. It so often turns to the dark side instead. It is crucial to survival to stay connected to others.

7. **The body ages, while the spirit matures.** There is no turning back the hands of time when it comes to the body. It will age. However, the eternal spirit inside of us matures. The body can, however, regenerate itself to a large extent if it is given enough energy. The brain is neuroplastic, meaning it can change if we have the intent to do so and provide the energy. Essentially, you *can* teach an old dog new tricks – if you give that dog enough energy.
8. **Sprints are better than marathons.** Just as with exercise, it is better to expend energy, take time to recover, then expend energy again, rather than trying to continually expend energy without rest. The human body needs sprints rather than marathons. It can fix itself in the breaks. Then it can sprint again. However, if we don't give it that ability to regenerate, it' likely to break. And that's no fun.
9. **We must learn to understand and appreciate others' love languages.** We are more powerful in connection with others, which means we must learn to understand how others express love. We need to be mindful of their sources of energy, which explains why they do what they do. Most times there is reason behind action. In understanding that reason, we can find forgiveness. And forgiveness is healing.
10. **Each individual has a body protector.** The job of the body is to protect the spirit within. If the body is low on energy, it will push others away to protect itself. Pushing others away for energy reasons is an objective, not an emotional, response. It is the body making a decision about how much energy it can expend and how. We just need to help others understand that we don't have the energy right now, not that we don't love them. Once we rejuvenate, we may be able to embrace what others need.
11. **Wellness is our responsibility.** No pill, medical professional or insurance company can give us wellness. It is our choice. Wellness extends beyond a colonoscopy or a

wellness exam. It is a state of mind committed to unification of the mind and body.

12. **The body views situational and biological stressors the same way.** Our body perceives stress arising out of situations and stress from biological dysfunction in the same way. Both put our spirit into a low power mode. So, if our thyroid is off, our body perceives this the same way as if there are tensions at home. And one may contribute to the other. Knowing this can help us understand that our life and our body are interconnected. We must fix our life to fix our body.
13. **Medication should be used to recycle your energy.** If we are given an aid such as medication to help get better, we should use its added power to recycle our energy. So, if it gives you relief, use that relief to process the stress or change your life, or else you may always need that medication. You have to give back to your body to enable it to recycle and power up again.
14. **If you don't fix the problem, your body will only accommodate you for so long.** You can cheat nature for a little by taking medication, skimping on sleep, etc. But ultimately if you do not fix the problem, your body will keep talking to you. And you may not like the message. So, for example, if you take an antidepressant but do not fix the source of the depression, you can get relief for a while. And then it's likely to stop working. Nature can beat any pill. It's up to you to figure out the "why."
15. **Aging is an opportunity to live more consciously.** Aging is an opportunity for the mature mind to give back to the body. Until about age 35, the body absorbs most of the blows of bad decisions. But after 35 or so, we start feeling the impact. Therefore, you have to learn to give back to your body more consciously so it can regenerate. The mature mind still has the power of the regeneration. It just takes more intention and care. The body is never against you. It always wants to help. Use the more mature mind to help it do so.

16. **Aging is an opportunity to let go of baggage.** As we age it becomes more important to let go of emotional baggage, which is heavy and weighs down the spirit. Carrying that weight long-term leads to a shorter life. So, decide for the sake of wellness to let it go – and live longer. I'm not saying this is easy. I'm just saying that it helps your journey. It is okay to let go and forgive. It doesn't mean what happened was right; it just means you are choosing to live a better life.

Chapter 4

Seven Premises of Wellness

When I turned 40, I had a few days of feeling down about it. It was the first time I started seeing myself on the other side of the aging curve. Then I reoriented my thinking to remember the people and things in my life that give me strength.

I reminded myself not to dwell on my body's battle wounds. I chose to see them as remembrances of the places I had been in my life.

I learned to let go of the thinking and practices that were holding me back and to pay more attention to taking care of myself. I had to remind myself to keep moving and to relieve stress. I had to learn to be very kind to myself, to deliberately give opportunities to my senses to reinvigorate me. I had to give my brain a hug of positivity. I had to embrace the potential of a new journey, to open my mind to the opportunities I had never explored, to be open to change. And I had to trust my intuition.

To this day, I find that the more I do all this, the less fearful I become. And chronic fearfulness is the essence of stress, which I believe is at the heart of many wellness issues.

We learn fear fairly early in life, at about the first grade. Before that, we look through the eyes of love, we are less competitive and we tend to help one another more. But when we enter a more structured societal environment, we start to worry about fitting in and what others think. We may override our body's fear response because of societal values, even if those values go against what our body is telling us (e.g., work harder instead of sleeping when we need it).

While we don't want to live by fear, we need to remember that fear is the power of nature trying to keep us alive and protect us. The brain needs energy to make decisions, and it will as a result choose the path that takes the least energy. The amount of energy in a decision is complex, depending upon our value system, the state of our body and many other variables. As we make these decisions, we need to learn to work with our body, rather than fight against it. We need to find the true power and freedom in peace. We need to learn to win by lifting others.

The mind is a powerful thing. Simply the way we think about things can cause significant biological changes. When we think that we are sick or when our minds perceive prolonged sadness or stress, we can physically get sick. And we can start to fear our fear.

I believe we can reduce our body's perception of stress so that we can return to a happy place. I believe this because I have done just that for myself. We need to unlearn the fear of fear, stop messing up our body's evolutionary compensatory mechanisms and stop trying to be society's model for desirability. Once you let go of whatever you are perceiving to be stress and the accompanying fear, your body forgives you and can rewire your brain. It literally is that simple – but anything but easy. Your brain can do this because it has amazing neuroplasticity, if it has the energy it needs. In fact, often the main thing I do with patients is help them unwind their fear response, which then helps their body unwind any metabolic dysfunction, including whatever is causing pain.

People are tired of being on the fear treadmill. They just don't know how to get off it. Once they learn how to remove the stressors that are preventing their bodies from fixing themselves, once they learn that every thought, experience and feeling matters as much as their genetic makeup, they can better work with me to identify any underlying pathologies.

Quite simply, chronic fear is unproductive. It just engenders more negativity, which disrupts our brain's neurotransmitters. One way to grasp this is to think of your body like a car. It generates exhaust (stress) each day. A large amount of exhaust ages us. If the muffler (output for stress) that releases that exhaust is clogged, the system will explode. But if the muffler is a big open pipe and the car is efficient, then the car keeps on rolling.

Like a car the body wants a good balance between stress taken in and stress relieved. As long as there is a balance of stress from within and from without (and this goes beyond situational stress to include aging, thoughts, biological function, etc.), then our spirit and our mind get to drive, or control, the body (our car, so to speak). But if we are out of balance for a long time, the body starts to drive or control the mind, lowering our metabolic rate to conserve itself, including its internal biochemical processes and the breakdown of substances. Quite simply, the brain would like something better than this.

As we gain understanding of the causes of our stress and how to relieve ourselves of it, we can be more proactive about our abilities to keep ourselves in balance – not just by medicine and supplements, but also by our other senses and our ability to be more intentional about our environment.

It is out of this thinking that I derived the following seven premises of wellness:

Seven Premises of Wellness

Premise 1: The brain naturally wants positive thoughts and to live in the present. But it takes energy to stay there. When the brain perceives something negative, it starts to problem solve. It wants the issue to go away. Oftentimes it looks to soothe itself through food, smoking, drinking or other means, in an attempt to find relief and try to make the sadness disappear. Over time, if we are not careful, we can gain a lot of weight, and our lives can become dysfunctional.

Premise 2: Our body lives by a rule book that is governed by thousands of years of evolutionary genetic adaptations. That rule book is primal and includes wanting to eat from the Earth, rather than from a diet of processed foods. It also includes a desire to move, which releases a lot of positive growth factors and neurotransmitters that help our brain and our body. We must alternate intensity with rest. We are not built to be marathoners who run all the time. Our stress response is built to sprint, then recover, then repeat that process.

Premise 3: We each have one body that is ours throughout our whole life's journey. We cannot change who we are. But we can maximize and optimize who we are. We need to accept how our body is structured. We can maximize our body by helping it be the strongest, leanest, most powerful that it can be. For instance, I am a mesomorph, built like a bulldog. I will never have a greyhound body, like the kind in the lingerie catalogues. I have learned to accept that. I hope you can do the same as regards your body. The alternative is a constant battle with your genetic composition. Long-term battling with how your body is made can make you sick.

Premise 4: If the brain is unhappy or the body is asked to do something that it is not made to do, this is perceived as stress. A stressed brain is a stressed body. If this is a chronic problem, the energy of the body will become imbalanced, causing even more stress. We must do what makes our brain happy and gives it energy. It is our computer.

Premise 5: The body perceives physical and emotional stress in the same way, so don't stress it in either way for prolonged periods.

Chronic physical and emotional stress is a recipe for a lack of wellness and potential disease. Allow for rest and recovery.

Premise 6: The stress hormone cortisol, our "fight or flight" hormone, is essential for life. It regulates how our body uses carbohydrates, fats and proteins; tamps down inflammation; regulates blood pressure; regulates blood sugar (the glucose in your system); controls our sleeping/waking cycle; boosts our energy to handle stress and then restores the balance afterward. Cortisol makes a lot of energy available to our muscles so they can move fast. It is a protective mechanism. Short bursts of it actually make us stronger. It is normal for the body to feel stress, so don't be scared of it. It is stress without adequate rest and recovery that is the problem.

Premise 7: Long-term cortisol production resulting from chronic stress makes us sick and leads to dysfunction. It is not normal for the body to go without a break. It wants to feel a certain amount of stress, then get a break before it feels it again. Chronic pumping of cortisol into our system can cause fear, irritability, unforgiveness, isolation and doubt about our life's value. What we are asking of our bodies in this day and age is not normal – they do not want to run an emotional marathon of emails, texts, phone calls, television, pressures, sitting and eating processed food. These are perceived as stress and continue to spike cortisol. That starts a cascade of bad events, such as increased body fat, difficulty remembering things, GI issues, trouble sleeping, anxiety and depression. Prolonged stimulation of cortisol through stress can actually lead to reductions in this hormone, which may skew how it is addressed medically. Basically, cortisol is not the issue. The real issue is the continued, elevated perception by the body that it is in a stressful environment, or in an environment that does not reconcile with its primal genome.

Given the chronic stress/fear response too many of us are experiencing and the results I see in my patients, I have come to see stress as the major problem of society. We need to address this, and here are ten tips as to how to do that:

10 Tips for Stress Reduction

1. Both children and adults are the least stressed in the morning hours. So this is the time to do the things you really don't want to do, especially if you are recovering from trauma.
2. Learn to take breaks and deep breaths and find some alone time a couple times a day. Take water breaks.
3. Don't give energy to what you cannot change.
4. Take time throughout your day for the little things that make you feel good, whether they be sights, sounds, smells or other enjoyable experiences, and give yourself to them freely.
5. Know how you compensate for stress, and take note of unhealthy tendencies (e.g., overeating). They are the first sign that your energy balance needs adjusting.
6. Do not condemn yourself for being in the rhino (acute) or bear (chronic) stress mode; just release the fear and have confidence that your body, mind and spirit can regenerate.
7. Try as much as possible to live in the present. If we spend our life thinking about the past or tomorrow, we forget to see today.
8. Check yourself when you hear negative comments about someone else coming out of your mouth – these adversely affect your stress and your health.
9. Don't feel you have to have everything all figured out. Your heart will guide you.
10. Never stop trying, believing and doing the best you can. Believe you are here for a reason and avoid wishing you were someone else.

Chapter 5

The Simple 7 Solution to Wellness

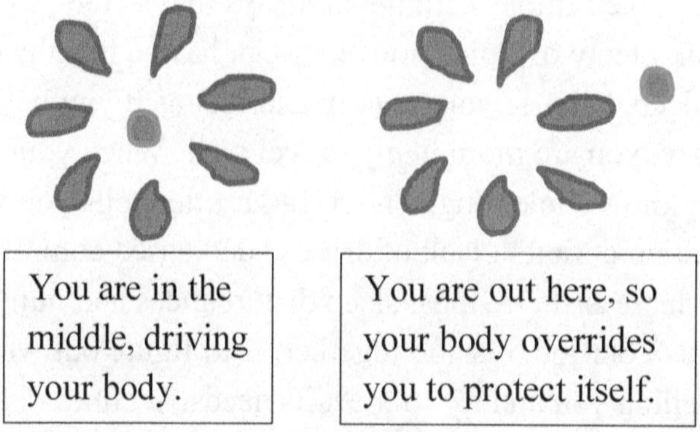

The seven petals in each of the illustrations above represent my seven rules for wellness, outlined in the Simple 7 principles discussed in this chapter. Examine each of them to see where you might be out of balance.

Out of my philosophy, I developed what I call the Simple 7 guide to wellness. And it is really all about energy conservation, balance and regeneration. At its essence it is about understanding your stress response and, where necessary, making adjustments in your spiritual, mental and physical well-being.

The Simple 7 is a framework of reference to listen to, and hear, what your body is telling you. As such, it's even more important to follow as your body ages and talks to you more. It is a reference point for you to learn what gives you energy so that you can achieve maximum wellness and continue regenerating your body, no matter what your age.

The Simple 7 is a simple concept, but it is not always simple to live by. However, it is a good place to start. It involves facing your demons that make you want to run away from your problems. It involves accepting and embracing yourself for who you are. And that can be hard.

Essentially, the Simple 7 framework says that as long as you eat well, drink plenty of fluids, move, sweat, have a healthy digestive system, sleep, balance your energy and feel as if you belong to a community, you are more likely to feel well. When your body wants to let you know something is not right, it often tells you with a concentration deficit, a lack of drive, a decreased commitment to exercise, increased cravings, sleep disturbances and numerous other indicators. Your job, our job together, is to figure out what your body is telling you and try to meet its needs. Wellness is all about helping unify your mind, body and spirit.

When it feels like something is not right in your body, analyze where in the Simple 7 you got off track, and try to correct that. If nothing has changed and you don't understand what's going on, that's when you should run an evaluation of your body, a diagnostic if you will. If you ask your body a question, it will tell you the answer. Your brain needs to understand why you feel the way you do. When it does, that leads to less worry and ultimately provides more energy to be well. In essence, if you can process "why" things are the way they are it is so much easier to let go of negative energy.

Simple 7 Principles

1. **Energy – Movement and Exercise**

Make moving a habit. Don't make it hard. Once you are consistently moving, mover smarter (not harder), incorporating strength and mobility exercises and making adjustments for age, injury, history, body type and life stressors.

How you move is how you de-stress. How you eat is how you lose weight. People often initiate movement before they change their diet. This can make sense because oftentimes we mix food with community, love and reward (if you take away or change food, the body looks at this as restrictive).

When we move more, we move stress away from our body, and this feels good. If you are in rhino mode (acute stress), running away can give you power. But remember not to run too long or you can break. If you are in bear mode (chronic stress), walking and doing yoga can relieve stress. Keep it up, and one day you will be walking and wanting to run, too.

In either case, your body is letting you drive, or give away energy. You are healing. You don't have to work out an hour a day. Every step counts. Every movement counts. Adjust your workout to your age. The older you get the tighter and less flexible you get. So mobility is even more important with age.

Be consistent. Don't make it too hard. Listen to your body. Adjust your workout. Learn to value strength and mobility.

2. Elements

We all need essential vitamins and minerals from the Earth. We should get as much as we can from food. But when our genes, our GI tract or the nutritional content of our food contribute to depletion, we need to supplement. Give your body what it needs to get better, and it can do great things.

It's best if we can get most of our vitamins and minerals from whole foods, but that's not always realistic. While you can go to the health food store and guess what supplements you need, you can just ask your body (meaning get blood work done so it can tell you what's missing).

If you are a high-performance athlete, you may need to supplement more because you use up so many elements to sustain your level of activity.

But ultimately you shouldn't take an excessive amount of supplements. Your body is always more powerful than a pill. You should take only what you need and what helps you feel better. I use regulated supplements so I know what's in them. When it comes to using herbal supplements as medicinal agents, it is important to know what to prescribe and how much. We do not want to overcompensate. And I should note here that we did not get any training about this in medical school. I've learned all I know through my practice, by testing what the body needs to get objective data and then, if necessary, making supplement recommendations and measuring the effects. Other necessary elements include drinking pure water to support cellular function and getting the right amount of sun (which supplies Vitamin D). These gives us energy and so much more.

3. **Esteem**

How you think about yourself is crucial to your physical, emotional and spiritual health.

It is important to your health that you believe you are here for a reason and that you matter. The odds are incredible that such a unique being as you would be created out of the potential combinations of millions of eggs and sperm. The likelihood that your unique self would have the opportunity to live is greater by far than your chances of winning the lottery. Quite simply, it is a miracle that the individual that is you was born at all. Let that sink in. It's a good reminder that we need to live in the present and have no doubt about our self-worth. If, as you age, you feel you are losing your sense of self, remember that you are now wiser and more confident.

Some people struggle with the appearance of their body as they age. I see sparks of self-empowerment after body sculpting, just as I see when someone has a breakthrough in self-empowerment. Patients feel more connected with themselves. Both give the body energy. Ultimately, we need to love ourselves for who we are. We need to listen to our body. It is our warrior to protect our unique selves. It has endless regenerative capacity, if given the opportunity. Pass that thinking on to your children.

4. **Eating**

We evolved in a cave, where we saw food as a fuel. Therefore we need to eat whole foods that our body understands. Don't make it hard.

We are primal beings, which means we need to primarily eat whole foods. This means shopping mostly from the outside aisles of grocery stores, where the less-processed food is featured. Choose an eating plan that you like and that is sustainable. Fad diets are just that – they come and go. Go light on fruits because they have a lot of sugar. It's okay to occasionally cheat, but try to be consistent. Intermittent fasting is okay, too.

As we age, our body and life in general, can get more stressful. We can get cravings at night – not because our willpower is low, but because we are tired. If you fix why you are tired, the cravings should go away.

Don't condemn yourself, thus thinking yourself into a worse state. That just gives energy to thoughts that don't change anything. Instead, put energy into an action plan that changes something. And remember, stressing your body by starving it is not the answer.

5. Equilibrium

We need a balance of energy in the mind and body, including between activity and rest. We need to stay in balance.

Equilibrium means balance. We need to stay in the driver's seat of our life, realizing that everyone has different energies, belief systems and experiences that require individual tweaking.

Our body generates energy within itself, gives energy away and takes energy from others. Each person has a finite amount of energy. The energy within us is the biological process that supports our body's function, including hormonal function, thyroid function, glucose metabolism and more, as well as the value we give ourselves. The energy we give away involves the part of us that we share with others, which we can think of as love or acts of service. The energy we take from others is the part of that others share with us.

Giving too much away at our own personal expense is not sustainable. The best example of this is caregivers' fatigue. We may feel at times that it is selfish to give to ourselves, but we have a biological need to do so. Only then can we truly help others. Energy that we take on from others may be painful, without our even knowing it (for instance, absorbing others' negativity or listening too much to their pain). Excesses of this can cause us to get sick because of the sensory and stimuli overload involved.

I see plenty of people during middle age, when the body starts aging and their reserve tanks of energy get depleted. They become aware that their body needs help. Here is where hormonal equilibrium is essential, as it affects mood, focus, sleep, sex drive, organ function and the accumulation of fat – for both men and women. Certain hormones can help our body recover, cope with stress and give us a feeling of control and calmness. We also need adequate sleep to ensure our body can recover.

Perhaps surprisingly, a major part of maintaining one's equilibrium is gaining understanding and feeling forgiveness. If the brain understands the *why* of something, it can make decisions and move on. If it does not understand *why*, it ruminates to try to find that answer, resulting in an endless expenditure of energy. The brain must reach a place of peace, where it can be calm even in the midst of noise, trouble and hard work. If we think we can solve a known problem instead of just thinking about it, then we can get where we want to go a lot easier with a lot less pain. As for forgiveness, you can think of this holistically as the brain needing to decide that the pain and energy of holding on to a thought is not worth it any more. It does not mean the experience wasn't painful or that we should negate the experience; it's just means that the brain would now like room for something better. It wants to reclaim the energy from what's been holding us back and put it toward living.

6. **Elimination**

To regularly eliminate waste and toxins, we need to pay attention to our gastrointestinal system, our ability to sweat, our intentional movement and how much water we drink.

Too many people have stomach pain, bloating, diarrhea, heartburn and chronic constipation. But we need to purge the toxins from our body by the regular, healthy elimination of waste. We also can detoxify by moving, sweating, liver detoxing and by taking saunas. A big part of healthy elimination comes from eating well, drinking enough fluids and exercising. A number of body functions participate in this – the liver, the gallbladder, the GI tract, the kidneys and the sweat glands.

Our liver detoxifies the blood, eliminating waste through the GI system, which is where 80 percent of your infection-fighting cells live. But the liver itself also may need detoxing from time to time. Think of it as an engine with gears. If the gears get too gooey, they won't work their best. Degrease or detoxify them and they do better.

The GI system, which includes the stomach, the small intestine and the large intestine, can get inflamed and bloated. And given the GI system's connection to the brain, this can cause us to feel forgetful and fuzzy-minded. Your GI tract and your brain come from the same layers of development. Therefore, if your gut is upset, so is your brain. Fix what is going on in your GI tract and you will likely think more clearly.

The kidneys filter the blood. They both eliminate what they filter and reabsorb what is needed by the body. They are very forgiving, but we can push them too far and damage them. It's important to keep our filters clean. Drinking enough pure water is one of the best ways, rather than loading up on sodas or other substitutes.

And finally, our sweat glands rid the body of toxins. Indeed, the skin is our body's largest organ. Sweating is a major mode of detoxification.

Sometimes we may feel like we have acid indigestion. But I am not a proponent of the chronic use of antacids because they mask the body's message that it doesn't like what we are eating or that we are under too much stress. Try to figure out why you have indigestion. For instance, heartburn can be a warning sign, like the engine light on your car. If you keep driving or tape over the warning light, there's still something wrong, even if you don't see it. Similarly, antacids, if chronically used to cover up indigestion, can stop us from digesting our food properly and can lead to a nutritional deficiency in the long-term. This can adversely affect our gut bacteria, leading to other problems.

I hear so much about probiotics. And I believe in them, but there is a lot more going on in your GI system that is important. While probiotics can be very helpful, they don't address the food allergies and sensitivities that are a significant issue for so many of us.

In all this, it's important to listen to the body and respond appropriately to help it heal. While our body would never try to hurt us, it can get confused. We need to figure out how to fix the source of the confusion and remedy it.

7. Engagement

You need to feel a sense of community, that you belong somewhere. It is crucial to your wellness and survival.

Having a sense of engagement in a community is essential. If there is disruption in our community, we also feel stressed. Community is not limited to fellow human beings; it can be whatever you feel community with (pets, nature, wherever you feel you belong).

Engaging in community does not mean subscribing to uniformity. Rather engagement with community means that we feel we belong to a place that celebrates our uniqueness, where we raise each other up and love each other for who we are. There is so much fear, protection, isolation and doubt in the world, when what we need instead is love, laughter, friendship, family, a sense of place and a sense of belonging. People need to touch more, interact more, listen more and look at each other more so they don't feel so alone. We are all connected, and we need each other. This is a biological fact. When our energies are in synchronicity, we experience endless beauty. When they are against one another, we experience pain and darkness.

Having a sense of community doesn't mean all confrontation is bad. Confrontation should be seen as an opportunity to work through a situation and hopefully lift each other up to a better place. We need to realize that we each have our points at times. And we need to more fully contemplate our words and actions. It is important to be aware and humble in our dealings with one another. We are weaker when we are fighting with one another, but we are stronger when our mind feels communally at peace.

In this world of electronics and artificial intelligence, we especially need to connect with one another to exchange energy. Computers and phones do not give us energy. They keep us from looking at each other and touching each other. They keep us from moving. They keep us from interacting with nature. They take away a lot of accountability for our words and actions. Civility is very important to connectedness. Our body sees incivility as dangerous. We are here to bring out the best in each other. As our inner spirit becomes aware of others' worth, fear begins to drop away. And we start to feel connected to everyone and everything. We achieve inner peace. We find endless potential.

Chapter 6

Conclusion

Your body has been talking to you your whole life. Have you been listening?

Never underestimate its power or that of the spirit it houses. Your body has the ultimate healing power and is built to heal itself, if given the opportunity.

I believe that wellness is all about embracing that journey. We don't have control over others or nature, but we have more control than we think over our mind, body and spirit.

The first third of life is about finding confidence in ourselves. The middle is about work, procreation or mastering a skill. And the last third is about pondering what it all has meant and coming to peace with our journey. Listening to our body becomes even more important as we age.

I want to remind you to keep in mind the importance of living in the present, of persistence, of love, of faith and of connection – because these are crucial to a successful wellness journey. Remember, true wellness is when your mind and body are in sync and you are honoring the uniqueness that is you, knowing that you share humanity with all.

Slow things down so you can be open to the messages that are there for you, so you can hear what your body wants. Presence is a peaceful place where each day is colorful and full of messages, if you are willing to see. You cannot look in the rear view mirror and be present. You cannot look too far forward and be present either. You have to look at now, at today.

At whatever age you are, whatever gender you are, remember that you matter. Take time for yourself and for your body's maintenance. Your body is your ultimate warrior, but you must listen to it.

Believe in yourself – and even in something more than yourself. Believe you are here for a reason and that you have nothing to prove to anyone. You were born perfect and beautiful. You are unique. Revel in that thought. Don't worry about being like everyone else or trying to fit in. Celebrate who you are. Know that you matter, that everything matters.

Never give up on your wellness journey. It is miracle enough that you are alive. It is a miracle that there can always be some measure of improvement. It something has changed, your body is telling you to fix it. Learn what you need to fix, and fix it. You have nothing to fear from your body. It is your guide, your friend, your protector, your warrior. See it that way, and learn to love it rather than fear it. Flood it with energy, and it will lift you to great heights. And remember, your body is so forgiving that you only have to get it a little right, according to its genetic rule book.

Often we fear failure, but there really is no failure in wellness. The only failure is in never trying to adjust your direction when needed. Or in giving up and sinking. Choose to try again, using the wisdom of the changes you have made. Choose to stand up for your wellness. Every time something does not go your way, think of it as a force guiding you to turn. There is no failure in learning, growing and adjusting; there is only accumulated knowledge of the unique person that is you who is seeking to satisfy your needs. You can only fail yourself. And if you feel you have done that, forgive yourself as your body forgives you.

Keep faith with that spirit that is within you and is leading you on your journey. Don't spend too much time wondering why that journey is both painful and joyful. Just keep centered and await the truth to be revealed to you in your heart, in your sleep, during a long walk and at the most unlikely times. It will come rushing at you when the time is right, which is not necessarily when you demand it. Trust in your own personal timeline.

Stay connected to other living creatures and to nature. We feed off one another. Our energies in synchronicity with others bring endless beauty; our energies in continual, unresolved cross purposes with others bring pain and darkness. We need to lift each other up in humility, believing that no one is better or more right than another. The goal needs to be a better outcome for all. We cannot achieve wellness in a vacuum. The human spirit craves positive connection. It does not want to be alone.

We need to take responsibility for the world we have created and its effect on our bodies. We have to reduce the stressors that cause imbalance and illness. Change takes energy and self-accountability. It takes recognizing the unique factors that affect us and the common factors we share.

Ultimately we should be able to think and move in a high-quality way until our last day on Earth. There is a finite amount of energy in the world, but whether it is more positive than negative is up to each of us. Making the world a better place starts with each of us. Every thought counts. Every moment counts. And as you add more positive thought to your life, the energy around you will change.

This journey has been one of the most painful and rewarding experiences for me. I have given up my classic community of medicine. But at the same time I have found complete love and forgiveness within my own family. And I have felt greater joy in helping my patients. Healing now is not just something that I was taught. Instead, what I was taught is a framework for understanding wellness. I now understand more from my heart than from my head. I am confident that everything in my life has happened for a reason. And it has brought me to where I am. I am thankful for all the joy and all the pain.

I am more than a doctor. I am a fellow human being with a lot of life experience, your teammate with the goal of lifting you up. And in lifting you up, we both get better.

Today, I am relentless in my pursuit of helping people feel love, presence and beauty that extends beyond the external. I commit myself to listening to you, to standing by you and to helping you figure things out. I have learned power from peace. I have learned where to give my energy. I find joy and self-worth in helping others find this place.

I truly believe in what I do. My body is guiding me to higher places. And my mind is astounded at times at that direction. I am letting go a little more every day of what I think I should be and what I learned, and just being who I am. It is energizing, at times terrifying, and harder even than medical school. I am leaving behind a world to which I won't be returning. While sometimes I feel like I am standing alone, I know that ultimately I am never alone. It is all part of an amazing journey that I am taking with you.

I am sure I am meant to be on this journey. It becomes clearer every day. But I cannot force the timetable or know what is around each corner. I just have to have faith in the journey, in knowing that every pain will someday bring me to a higher place. I have to just let it be. I hope I can help you see this, trust in it and believe it. I hope to give you a different perspective on wellness. I hope I can help restore that flicker of light back into your eyes. It is the reason I do this. And it is intoxicating. I love seeing that light come on. It is contagious.

Life is about more than surviving. It is about living. It is about a journey with twists and turns, peaks and valleys. This story – the story of you – is being written this very minute.

I've written this to help your journey be less painful and more beautiful, to help you understand your warrior self and to listen to it. Don't lose faith. Don't feel alone. Believe in your wellness. Believe in your power. Don't fear aging because your body has endless regenerative capacity. I tell patients all the time that life's journey is hard, but your body is actually easy. You can sculpt it and regenerate it if you work with its rule book.

Wellness does not start with medicine. It starts with the idea that it is okay to be you, whoever you are. I accept you as you are. And that is the most powerful thing that I can do to help you get better. In the process, I am a better person myself.

I went to medical school thinking I was learning how to heal people because doctors are supposed to fix things. But I have learned I went to school to better understand the human body. Now I am an educator and a voice from your body to you. So often you are your own healer. And it is my job to teach you how to do that. You have ownership of your health. And you have to want it.

I wish you peace and happiness in your journey toward wellness, a journey I myself am on. I hope to have the privilege of traveling with you.

Made in the USA
Monee, IL
04 November 2026

67378021R00036